Diabetes Solution

*by Your Concise Guide with Everything You Need
to do NOW to Keep Diabetes Under Control*

Copyright © 2016

Table of Contents

Introduction

So, you have been diagnosed with diabetes. Diabetes can affect your life in a very adverse way if you don't take the right action now. Did you know, for example, that this illness can increase your chances of suffering a stroke? What about a heart attack? It can also affect areas of your life that you may not even have thought of. Your sex life, your digestion, and even your bladder can be affected by diabetes when it is not kept under control.

This guide has been written to help you to do the best you can to keep diabetes in the background of your life, enabling you to live a productive and happy life, regardless of the presence of diabetes. Once you have it under control, it no longer has you in its grasp. Don't become a victim, only because you hadn't realized the implications of the diagnoses given to you by your doctor. The information in the book is written to help you to understand, in simple terms, what your diabetes means to you and how you can take the driving seat.

Your kidneys need you to do a little more work than you normally do, to ensure that they are not expected to deal with excess waste, provoked by ignoring your illness. You can suffer from eyesight impairment and even foot disorders if you are not able to take the disease seriously. I have put all this bad news in the introduction. Your doctor has probably advised you of the risk factors, though it is necessary that you appreciate how serious these are. The good news is that we have devoted the rest of the book to the positive aspect of taking control of your diabetes.

You will need to make sure that your family understands the significance of your illness so that they can work with you on keeping it under control. Spell out the dangers so that they help you to take your lifestyle seriously. A group effort really will help you to stick to the guidelines provided within the pages of this book. You will also need specialist help at some stage, though this is detailed in the book so that you can be aware of changes in your body which may need to be dealt with along the way. If you do this promptly, you will find that you can take control, and that's critical. Follow the chapters of the book – read it over and over until you know the information by heart, and then move on to being able to live with your diabetes in a lifestyle that suits both you and it – a way of life that doesn't have to be as restricted as you think!

Back Up

You will need the support of a regular practitioner, but it's also useful to make an appointment with a specialist in diabetes so that they can look at your notes and come up with a life plan that will help you. While we have detailed a life plan that will work for diabetes, your specialist will know your particular details, and it's vital to have regular check-ups so that you are aware of the evolution of the illness.

You may notice changes in your body that need to be looked at from the beginning, such as changes in your digestive pattern, the health of your feet and any deterioration in your eyesight. Thus, once you have been diagnosed, visit an eye specialist and have a check-up as this gives you something to measure future results against should your eyes become affected. A foot specialist or chiropodist should also examine your feet at the beginning of your treatment so that comparisons can be made when looking for any potential changes.

By visiting these specialists, you are setting up markers and learning more about your diabetes at the same time. The markers can be used when you suffer any potential changes because the doctors will be able to see those changes straight away and this helps to limit the inconvenience of diabetes.

You will also need to invest in a blood sugar meter, and your doctor will be able to show you how to take readings and how to understand the significance of these readings. These measure the glucose levels in your body from a single drop of blood and are not hard to use. The standard for you will be told to you by your doctor, although in general, the average glucose level for most people (taken first thing in the morning and before meals) is between 70 and 130, rising to 180 or less after you have eaten. Women who are pregnant need to know that the ideal reading is between 60 and 99 and that a reading two hours after eating should be at the lower level of less than 130. If you have developed diabetes while you are pregnant, it is important to discuss the figures with your specialist so that you know what numbers you are aiming for.

It is important to make a chart and keep this with you at all times, showing the numbers as this helps you to make important decisions about what you eat, what physical activity you are capable of and how much of your medicines you are in need of. Bear in mind that you do need to have a clear medicinal plan worked out with your doctor in advance and that you should adhere to the instructions the doctor gives you.

If you have a cell phone, it's a splendid idea to download an app that allows you to record your readings. An electronic tracking system lets you have this information with you at all times which means that if you do suffer at any time, you can merely show the treating doctor what your problem is. By doing this, you are ensuring that you are safe, and that's an important part of care.

The other people you need to get onboard with your illness are your family and friends. Although it may be a joke to them that eating the wrong kinds of things is naughty, it means more than that to you. If you have friends and family understanding your predicament, you are much more likely to be able to stick to a plan which will help you to control your diabetes for life. These are people who care about you, and when you don't have sufficient willpower, they will be able to bring you back into line. Sometimes a problem shared helps you to keep on the right track.

Your family should know, for example, about the signs that may happen when you suffer from hyperglycemia. You may show evidence of weakness or become very thirsty. You may find yourself urinating more often than normal. Your attention span may be affected. Yeast infections are also another side effect of hypoglycemia. Let your relatives know the exact position because they will be able to help you when you are not able to help yourself. Remember, the idea is to keep the numbers in line with the guidelines given earlier, and you will find that creating a pattern to your life will help you to keep those numbers steady. If your relatives and friends know the bare bones of the illness, they will be able to help if and when your readings are high. In the early days, before you have found your feet, you may find that this happens – but it's nothing to be too concerned with. All you need to do is visit your doctor and show him/her the readings so that your treatment can be adjusted or they can reinforce ways in which you can bring those levels back down again.

Similarly, if your levels are too low, you can feel extra hungry or may get a little shaky. You can also get quite confused, so make sure that your family knows about this possibility in advance so that they don't panic when and if it happens. This is called hypoglycemia and in the worst case scenario you may pass out. If this happens, your family should call 911 immediately. However, this information is only given so that you know both ends of the scale and can manage your diabetes better, knowing the potential seriousness of ignoring what your body is trying to tell you.

Dealing With Low Glucose Situations

Some people are overly cautious when they are first diagnosed with diabetes. They see it as a potentially life-threatening illness when it doesn't have to be and they over-react, which may lead to low glucose. If this happens, there are things that you can do to bring the level back into the acceptable parameters.

It is a good idea to have a supply of glucose gel, which you can purchase at your local pharmacy. It's also a great idea to have glucose tablets because these are already measured into doses – meaning that you don't have to worry about that side of it. Three glucose tablets can help you get those figures back up again, and you will be feeling better within no time at all, although if your levels are very low, you can take four. In the case of glucose gel, you will find that the measurements are clearly marked on the pack, and you will need only one serving to try to bring your levels back to normal.

If you don't have any of these in the house, then a soft drink can help you to stabilize, and this should avoid diet drinks as they don't have the same glucose strength as other soft drinks and at this time, you need glucose. Sugar or honey can do the same thing, so even if caught out while you are in a restaurant, you can correct the situation by taking a spoon of sugar or honey to help the glucose rates to rise.

One friend of mine carries hard candies in her handbag at all times and swears by them as being her "lifesavers", and it's a pretty easy way to deal with having low glucose. If it is only marginally low, she takes two or three hard candies. However, if it looks like the numbers are drastic she eats up to six and says that she finds her levels come back to normal very quickly.

The chances are that if you get yourself into a situation where your levels are low, you will be alerted to it by apathy and tiredness. When this happens, take a reading. If the reading is low, sit down in a quiet place and take whatever your choice of remedy is. Allow it to enter your bloodstream and a way of doing this can be to take a very slow walk in a safe environment. If you are in a busy shopping mall and find that your levels are so low you are panicking, stay seated and wait for a little while. As soon as the levels improve, you will find that your body feels back to normal.

It sounds fairly scary, but you get used to your body's response to life and do get a fairly good idea that something is amiss, giving you time to deal with it. If this means carrying a few sugar cubes or hard candies with you at all times, then it's better than having to search for something to help your levels – especially when you are in a strange environment. After about 15 minutes, you need to check your levels again to see if they have improved. They should improve within this time, but if they need a further boost, take whatever is your choice of remedy once again to make sure that your glucose levels are within acceptable parameters.

Letting people know what's wrong

If your family and friends are aware of your diabetes, they will be a lot more understanding if symptoms occur. It doesn't have to be a traumatic situation. You may even want to buy yourself a bracelet so that medical staff will know what the problem is if your levels get so low that you cannot respond. Tell your family about what to do in a situation such as this. It's not like you are asking them for anything medical. You simply need them to understand that your levels are bottoming out and that you need to take in sugar in one of the formats shown above to get yourself back to your normal self.

Kenny is a diabetic and quite frequently at the beginning of treatment, he panicked. When his levels changed, he telephoned his doctor. When they were too high, he panicked even more than when they were too low. "If people had been straight with me from the beginning," he said, "I would simply have carried hard sweets with me for lows, and I would have been able to take control. However, what happened was that I didn't know the potential symptoms and thus, when they happened, had no idea how to control diabetes. It scared me."

Kenny is now fully in control of his diabetes. He laughs at his earlier attempts to seek medical help and thinks his doctor must have seen him as a hypochondriac at times. The time when you need to contact a doctor is when you believe you are not in control and perhaps your medicinal treatment may need to be adjusted. You can't do that. However, you can control the low glucose quite easily, so this chapter should have taken that worry out of your mind.

Understanding Blood Pressure Problems and AIC Readings

AIC readings and what they are used for

AIC readings are readings done by your doctor or specialist to determine your percentage of glucose over a set period of the last three months. This is a diagnostic test done by a physician. It's nothing to worry about because it's a simple pinprick to take a sample of blood but it gives your doctor an awful lot of information about you, which is essential to the treatment plan that you are on. Ask your doctor or your specialist how often this test needs to be done and mark it down on your agenda so that you don't leave it to chance. It's a great indication to the doctor as to whether your handling of diabetes, together with any medication, is working. You may find that your AIC reading shows the doctor that you are looking after yourself and keeping your glucose levels within acceptable parameters, and that's good news – rather than bad – so don't think of the test as being something to worry about. It's a precaution.

Why it's important to understand your blood pressure

Your blood pressure determines the amount of work that your heart has to do to pump blood around your body. If your blood pressure is too high on a consistent basis, this puts strain on the heart and people with diabetes need to try to keep their blood pressure below 140/80. However, your doctor is the only one who can advise you what the correct pressure is for you, bearing in mind your background.

DIABETES SOLUTION

When you have diabetes, you can help keep diabetes under control by taking regular exercise. This helps the blood flow and is the best way to ensure that you keep your blood pressure normal. If you have been a bit of a couch potato, don't worry. A short walk with the dog each day will help you to build up to longer walks. Don't suddenly become the Marathon Man! When you exercise, it takes a little while for you to get accustomed to that exercise. One thing that is known is that exercise promotes energy. When you exercise for the first time, you may not feel that this is the case, but as you learn to incorporate gentle exercise into your life, you will begin to feel a lot more energized, and that helps you to keep control of your blood pressure.

Swimming is another cardiovascular workout that is non-impact, so it's suitable for people even if they have problems with their feet and cannot walk far.

How to keep your cholesterol in check and why you need to

Cholesterol (the bad kind) can clog up your arteries and lead to heart disease. Your blood cannot flow as smoothly as it would had you not eaten the wrong kinds of foods or had habits that encourage blood clotting. Smoking is one area you can do something about. Even if you can't give up, try nicotine replacement. However, the cholesterol levels usually indicate that there is something in your diet that needs to be changed. One thing you can do if your cholesterol levels are borderline is eat a couple of apples a day. Some doctors prefer this route to statins because drugs can often have side effects that make the patient feel worse. In the next chapter, we will talk about diet options for diabetics, and this will also cover the foods that are helpful in controlling your cholesterol levels as well as telling you which foods to exclude.

Things that you can do to help yourself are to read labels and avoid things that are heavy in sugar content. For example, if you want to eat fruits, be aware that too much fruit may have too much sugar content. These are not obvious things, although you should avoid freshly squeezed orange juice because this actually will send your body into overload.

In the next chapter, we will deal with foods you can eat and those that you cannot. We will also outline things that you need to know about why you should avoid different foods that you may currently enjoy. It's not about control. It's about finding enjoyment in other foods than the ones that you are accustomed to, and there are some great foods out there that will help to lower cholesterol and are not as bland as you may suppose.

Foods to Avoid and Why

Your doctor will have already given you a diet sheet showing you the foods that are encouraged. There may also be a note of the foods to avoid, but you may not know the significance of why you need to avoid them. It helps you to keep your diabetes under control if you do know this because it gives you more incentive to stay within the set parameters, and thus keep your diabetes under control.

Carbohydrates – This includes foods such as bread, pastries, and cakes. Yes, I know exactly what you are thinking but which would you rather? High glucose levels that threaten your health or excellent health and the ability to live a relatively easy life? If you load on the carbohydrates, you are using up the calories that you could use to supply yourself with great nutritious meals that are delicious. They can also mean that you slow down your metabolism and won't want to do exercise. That's bad news for a diabetic. Accept that this is something that is life threatening and avoid it. You will be able to find replacements and food habits are just that – habits. When you get into healthy habits, you will find equally attractive things.

Fats – Excess fat and grease help to clog up the arteries. Since you already have diabetes, it's vital to keep your cholesterol levels down to live a reasonable life. Choose meats that are low in fat because they are equally delicious. Chicken and white meats are great to eat as well as fish – but leave out the batter! There are so many different types of fish to choose from, and you will find yourself developing a whole new eating experience and loving every minute of it. Introduce new fish a little at a time until you know which ones you feel good about eating. Fats will kill you. That's good enough reason to keep in control of what you eat.

French Fries - This may be a hard one at first to accept. However, when you see what French fries contain – even the low fat varieties are a bad choice for people with diabetes. Avoid them. Try new potatoes steam baked with mint. You will find that the taste is excellent and that there are no hidden ingredients. French fries in a restaurant situation can hide so many things. Calories, total fat, saturated fat, sodium, and carbohydrates are the ones that instantly come to mind.

Bought biscuits and cookies - During the manufacturing process, you have to remember that foods such as this are made tempting to the consumer intentionally. They are also loaded with the kind of ingredients a diabetic needs to avoid. Instead of eating these, look out for recipes for diabetic cookies. At least you will know what is in them, and you will gain the pleasure of sharing them with the family – lessening their chances of becoming diabetic as well.

In a restaurant situation

Many of the foods that are dangerous to diabetics are hidden in restaurant prepared food. You may think that the nacho on your plate looks delicious and nutritious but don't be fooled by healthy presentation. A nacho can contain more than 850 calories and if you want to add any dressing – forget it! Read the menu carefully and go to trusted restaurants where you know fresh ingredients are used, and healthy choices are available. You would be better, for example, to have a serving of duck rather than a serving of a convenience food. Duck is excellent for you and presents good cholesterol. Opting for grilled fish instead of battered fish is a great option, and you can ask for a salad without dressing, but make it more enjoyable by choosing one that has a variety of ingredients such as avocados, tomatoes, cucumber, different types of lettuce and onion. If you need a dressing opt for olive oil based dressings rather than those that are based on other oils that are less healthy alternatives. In fact, Olive Oil and vinegar make perfect dressings that don't kill the taste of the food. Add a zest of lemon to give your salad that extra lift that you need.

For a desert, be aware that restaurants are now in the habit of offering stylized coffee. You'll want to avoid this because of hidden ingredients. Avoid full cream ice cream and opt for fruit salad or even fresh salad. If you choose fruit salad, check with the counter staff that the salad is not a processed one from a can because this hides so much sugar content that it would be against the rules to eat it. It's your body, and you need to be aware of your choices. Be careful to measure your glucose levels as well, as these may reveal that you have eaten something that contained something you were not aware of. It's important to find restaurants that offer great food that isn't disguised. Fast foods are off the menu.

In a restaurant situation, avoid fruit juices and cordials. At home, you can control the level of added sugar by buying the best for your condition – avoiding orange juice that contains too much concentrated sugar. Sodas hide sodium, and that's equally bad for you. Learn to drink more water because when you do, you will find that your body will thank you for it. Although people don't admit to not drinking enough fresh water, clean water can help you to overcome many of the hurdles faced by individuals who are a little overweight and who have not exercised sufficiently. It helps to keep your body hydrated, and your muscles supple. Coffee – although made with water – doesn't do the same thing.

Changing Your Eating Plan

If you have ever sat down to a large meal and then felt that awful fatigue afterward, you will know that this is a situation that you need to avoid as a diabetic. It's a sign of eating too much all at the same time. You need to get into the habit of eating small amounts but on a regular basis. The idea is to keep the glucose levels the same all the way through your day and night so that you do not suffer. In fact, those who have adopted an eating plan that includes small snacks mid-morning and afternoon, as well as smaller meals that are controlled in calorie content, have found they can live relatively normal lives and keep their diabetes under control.

You will need to make sure that your kitchen is stocked with plenty of things you can eat so that you can make excellent snacks and light meals without having to go through the temptation of shopping every five minutes. Instead of buying white bread, get yourself some whole grain bread and even brown pittas, as these are helpful for creating a lunchtime meal that isn't too high in calories. Remember, you have a list you can refer to from your doctor, but there are some things you need to remember:

Vegetables – The brighter the color, the more useful the food. Bell peppers are excellent and the red ones taste lovely. Green vegetables such as spinach are healthy, and you can be inventive with vegetables of this nature. Ever tried an omelet made with spinach? It's very delicious. Frozen vegetables are a great aid to quick food preparation, but avoid those that are already made into meals because they will contain all kinds of things that are bad for you. If you insist on eating potatoes, cut down the amount and enjoy new potatoes in season – sprinkled with mint. Get used to using a steamer because this helps you to keep the flavor locked in.

Fruit – These make ideal snacks. What's wrong with an apple and a few raisins? It beats eating things that are unhealthy. Remember that if you do juice fruit, avoid juicing oranges because these do produce an overload of sugar.

Protein foods – You need these for healthy growth. Boil eggs, as these are a wonderfully flexible friend when it comes to making meals such as salads or pittas. Chicken and tuna are also high-value sources of protein. If you make sure that your larder is filled with healthy alternatives, you may find that your kids will follow suit. Try to get rid of all of the problematic foods so that you are not tempted. If you insist on eating chocolate, buy it from a health food store and allow yourself small portions. Diabetic chocolate can also be used to make your desserts more enjoyable.

Your food doesn't have to be boring. However, you do need to plan your meals and make sure that you have the ingredients ready to provide your body with the fuel it needs. You will get accustomed to its needs and will find, as you do, that you will also get accustomed to new tastes and temptations along the way. Recently Katy, who has been diabetic for three years, discovered yellow kiwi fruit and found this to be a real treat to stop her from getting tempted to eat sugared or carbohydrate dense foods as snacks.

The main rule of thumb for diabetics is that you can have "all of the things you choose from your approved list in moderation." It wasn't moderation that brought you to being diagnosed with diabetes, and now you need to exercise control over your eating habits and will find it entirely possible to live a very healthy lifestyle if you can keep to the rules.

Super fruits that help to keep glucose levels down

When I mention the names of these fruits, remember what we said about all things in moderation. You cannot simply pig out on these foods, but you can add them to your daily intake, and they will help you to stay on track, as well as giving you a real treat. One orange a day is sufficient which is why we do not recommend making orange juice. It is helpful to eat an orange because it contains soluble fiber, which makes sluggish digestion more efficient. Watermelon reduces the level of glucose, and although it's had a bit of bad press for containing sugar, this isn't the case. Enjoy it. Pears and apples also have fiber that helps digestion, but they also help with circulation, as well as being able to help cut cholesterol. Guava, avocado, and kiwis also contain vitamins and minerals but are rich in fiber so are helpful in your diet.

You can control your diabetes yourself. It's all a matter of adjustment. Drink enough fresh water and avoid bottled water unless contained in glass containers. Get enough rest as that provides the body with a natural system of healing. Make sure you don't skip meals and to ensure you are not caught out in situations where the only food available is unsuitable, get used to carrying your food around in a refrigerated box so that you have choices.

Conclusion

When people think of the word "diabetes" they instantly think of restriction. However, rational thought about what you eat will keep your blood glucose levels in check. You will find that you will develop new habits that are equally rewarding and will acquire the taste for great food. The AIC test tells your doctor how hard you are trying and if you ensure that you adhere to the rules, you will find that your body will thank you for the difference you make to its function.

As with all illnesses, these are cries from the body to do something different to your habitual actions and deeds. Perhaps the best thing about getting diabetes under control is the fact that your body will become much more capable of handling life. You will have more energy than you remember having before and with regular exercise and drinking of fresh water, will feel like you are younger.

Don't forget your regular checkups because these are what keep you in control of your health. You may find that if you are super-sensible, you will be able to limit the amount of medication that you need and can thus avoid all the side effects as well. Never change your dosage without consulting your doctor. It is the results of tests that will determine any changes.

People can live for years with diabetes. It's the body's way of saying "enough is enough." When you start to listen to your body and can keep your glucose levels regular, you will also find that your chances of heart disease and stroke are diminished because of the action you take to prevent a diabetic crisis. That's got to be good news, and when your blood test comes back with good news, you will know that you have indeed kept your diabetes under control.

Bonuses! Free Stuff For you!

If You Want Free Best Selling Kindle Books Delivered to Your Inbox on a Weekly Basis

Head over to http://liveyourdreams.guru/free-kindle-book-club/

As a way of saying thank you for your purchase I am giving you an additional ebook FREE!!   You can download this free ebook now! Simply head over to http://liveyourdreams.guru/diabetes-solution/

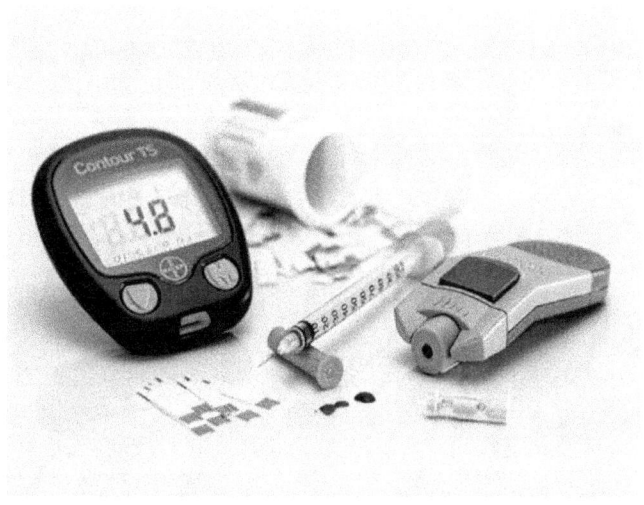

www.ingramcontent.com/pod-product-compliance
Lightning Source LLC
Chambersburg PA
CBHW070310190526
45169CB00004B/1568